DEFEATING DENTAL ANXIETY

DR. CHI MBA

Copyright © 2021 Dr. Chi Mba.

All rights reserved. No part of this book may be reproduced, stored, or transmitted by any means—whether auditory, graphic, mechanical, or electronic—without written permission of the author, except in the case of brief excerpts used in critical articles and reviews. Unauthorized reproduction of any part of this work is illegal and is punishable by law.

ISBN: 978-1-7162-8312-3 (sc)
ISBN: 978-1-7162-8311-6 (e)

Because of the dynamic nature of the Internet, any web addresses or links contained in this book may have changed since publication and may no longer be valid. The views expressed in this work are solely those of the author and do not necessarily reflect the views of the publisher, and the publisher hereby disclaims any responsibility for them.

Any people depicted in stock imagery provided by Getty Images are models, and such images are being used for illustrative purposes only. Certain stock imagery © Getty Images.

Lulu Publishing Services rev. date: 12/23/2020

Table of Contents

INTRODUCTION	vii
CHAPTER 1	1
The Deadly Fear	1
What is dental anxiety?	1
People who are afraid of dental appointments	2
CHAPTER 2	5
The discovery	5
Causes of dental anxiety	5
Signs of Dental anxiety	7
Effects of dental anxiety	10
The risk of not overcoming dental anxiety	14
CHAPTER 3	17
Oral health	17
Dental problems	18
Causes of dental problems	20
How to maintain proper dental hygiene	22
CHAPTER 4	25
Dental visitations	25
Expectations vs. reality	25
Why people should visit the dentist	28
When should we visit the dentist?	30

Managing dental anxiety during dental appointments	31
The next big thing for the people who visit the dentist	33
CHAPTER 5	**37**
The Dentist's Corner	37
Effective ways to handle patients with dental anxiety	38
CONCLUSION	**41**

INTRODUCTION

Sweets are lovely, desserts are good, but when it's time to see a dentist, these things aren't fun anymore. While some people enjoy going to the dentist, many people feel a great deal of anxiety about it. As a result of fear, many have avoided dental checkups completely. 80 percent of humans experience dental phobia. Dental phobia can take many forms. Often, there is a general fear of allowing things to come close to the teeth. Some people have a deep distrust of dental appointments. Dental phobia also varies in its intensity. Although some people have a slight doubt, others are terrified of dental visits. When an individual is very terrified of dental visits, it will prevent them from getting adequate professional care. This fear, in all of its variations, may have severe consequences for an individual's oral and general health. The result of dental phobia is known as dental evasion, leading to bad oral health. Dental anxiety has been shown to play a critical role in resisting treatment and care.

The irony is that, as a result of dental anxiety, many people flee from reality. Dental fear facilitates an unsafe oral lifestyle. Exceptionally high dental anxiety can affect one's quality of life. In most cases, when people ignore their oral care, it can lead to low self-esteem. Developing a little concern about dental visits may be normal. However, seeing the dentist is equally as important as a regular physical checkup. A healthy lifestyle without healthy oral health isn't complete. Some people who refuse to go for dental checkups report that they are afraid of the "tools" used by the dentist. Others complain that dentists are not responsive and warm to people. I will attempt to respond to some of these concerns.

This book expresses the need to resolve dental distress by illustrating the need for appropriate dental treatment, the importance of dental appointments, and identifying how to recognize dental anxiety. We will examine symptoms and sources of dental anxiety as well as identifying the need for dental appointments and different approaches to ensure that dental visits are manageable and effective. My earlier book "Overcoming Dental Anxiety" was written as a workbook to help address the issue and give the patients tools to identify their problem. This book is written to provide more in depth information and to accompany the workbook. It is important to acknowledge that dental anxiety is a concern for specific individuals. It is worth mentioning that although I am a dentist, I also experience a form of dental anxiety. I can relate from both sides of the aisle. You've come across this guide because you need a solution to your dental distress, so let's dive in!

CHAPTER 1
The Deadly Fear

What is dental anxiety?

Fear is generally characterized as a person's reaction to an immediate danger occurrence or an unsafe circumstance to save one's life. Typically, the answer to fear is to flee. We have common worries, and we always want to get away from them. Some people consider their fear of the dentist as their worst fear. Dental anxiety is a dangerous paranoia that can do a lot more harm than good to an individual. It is the powerfully negative emotions associated with dental treatment in infants, teenagers, and adults. Dental anxiety leads to stress, pressure, or discomfort in a dental environment. Being frightened to see a dentist can result in resisting or refusing dental treatment. The aforementioned paranoia is indeed dangerous, for it hinders safe living and can affect an individual's overall existence. Poor oral hygiene can lead to a slew of other medical problems. Dental anxiety can lead to negative responses to dental treatment. This response is capable of causing problems for both the dentists and the patient involved. Dental stress is a normal emotional reaction to one or more particular hazard factors in a dental setting. Dental anxiety, though, suggests a state of fear that anything wrong could happen during dental care, which is generally followed by a sense of lack of control. Dental phobia is a state of heightened anxiety that may include anxiety of dental procedures, the dental atmosphere or the setting, fear of dental equipment, or fear of the dentist. People with dental phobia frequently avoid seeing the dentist and neglect their oral hygiene, which may lead to severe dental complications and eventually cause them to visit the dentist in an emergency nature. In this emergency state, their treatment may become more aggressive which can raise their phobia. It is easier to get a dental cleaning than to get a tooth extracted. Most people with dental anxiety only show up for extractions and root canals. The influence of this phobia goes as far as causing stress in relationships and negatively influencing career lifestyle, social life, and interactions.

Dental phobia is a real occurrence. And it can have significant health effects if it is permitted to interfere with dental treatments or visits. It can also lead to multiple health problems such as acute physical impairment, drowsiness, fainting, or shortness of breath, However it can be managed by giving a proper setting and a knowledgeable dentist. You deserve to be well, and a lot of good health starts from your mouth. However, it is necessary to recognize dental phobia and to know how to cope with it… And there is a solution.

People who are afraid of dental appointments

Dental anxiety affects people of all ages. Many people have dental anxiety; therefore, you are not alone. Data indicates that dental anxiety is widespread globally and is not limited to a community or region. 5-20 percent of people suffer from extreme dental anxiety. It is estimated that 80 percent of Americans have some dental anxiety and 5-14 percent have severe dental anxiety. Many researchers have discovered that dental anxiety is more common in women. This is partly because they are more likely to come to the dentist and more likely to show their emotions. Dental anxiety has also been reported to decrease with age. Research indicates that older patients feel less pressure during dental procedures. A study has revealed that past painful experience is an essential initiating factor in dental distress and anxiety. Children who have had bad dental experience in most cases will overcome their concerns if the condition is appropriately handled, they are adequately cared for, and they are encouraged during subsequent dental visits.

In some cases, individuals who develop dental phobia do so because of their painful encounters with the dentist. Some people need to hear the sound of a hand piece to trigger that pool of sweat. Studies suggest that between 48% and 60% of the population have a form of anxiety or fear of dental treatment. There is also a small percentage of people who have dental anxiety for unknown reasons. Many of these individuals may or may not have anxiety in other areas of their lives.

CHAPTER 2
The discovery

Causes of dental anxiety

Dental anxiety is capable of provoking uneasiness. People with dental distress get a feeling of unease over upcoming dental consultations. They may also have exaggerated doubts or suspicions. Dental phobia is a more extreme disorder that makes people panic-ridden and afraid. People with dental phobia are mindful that their apprehension is entirely unfounded; however, they are powerless to do anything to alter it. It is usually a period of flight or fight for them. Different individuals convey varying types of dental distress. Several approaches have been developed to alleviate anxiety and dental panic. In addition to the diagnosis and management of dental anxiety, various types of dental anxiety have been identified. The fear of dental appointments is induced and always with a cause. However, the reasons for dental anxiety are as complex and diverse as the people who feel it. Various factors cause it, and the common factors include:

1. Quickly established phobia — fear of dental procedures: The thoughts of dental operations alone can lead people to cancel dental appointments. Many people are terrified of tools and instruments used by the dentist. The sight of these machines causes discomfort that leads to uncontrollable fear. For certain people, only the sound of the hand piece could lead to a severe anxiety attack. Dental anxiety is conveyed when this terror comes to action.

2. Fear of disaster: There is a concern that something might go wrong or that dental operations might not go as anticipated. Dental anxiety may be expressed in fear of physical health crises, such as panic attacks, heart attacks in adults, and even fainting. One can accurately diagnose dental fears when a patient spontaneously demonstrates a panic attack. Panic attacks can also lead to further issues.

3. Fear of pain: Some people may have had a traumatic dental experience in the past culminating in their fear of pain. Certain dental operations may be uncomfortable, but you still have a range of choices to alleviate discomfort. Dental anxiety can be easily identified through the fear of pain, which could be boldly written on a patient's face.

4. Generalized anxiety — the naturally anxious individual: While anxiety is a large part of our life, some people are excessively anxious. When it's time for dental appointments, those people tend to overthink the dental procedures. Panic and physical reactions continue to rise while they're in the dental environment. It is usually evident in their countenance, and they can't hold back their fear.

5. Previous traumatic experiences: Past encounters are the basis for the future. When one has a painful dental procedure, dental distress is likely to arise. The human being instinctively rejects discomfort and does not like to go through more pain. Horrible dental experience can contribute to a dental phobia. Any time the patient recalls the level of pain, tension occurs.

6. Trust issues: Some people have general confidence problems that make them cynical and terrified of the unknown. They don't trust the dentist's words, no matter how much he/she claims, 'you're going to be great; it's not going to hurt.' This

anxiety is often related to previous traumatic experiences when their trust had been broken once. They no longer want to go through extreme pain.

7. Fear of the dentist: Many people are hesitant to have dental treatment and terrified of the dentist. This may be due to a negative experience in the past, or the impression that dentists like inflicting discomfort. Many dread the sight of a dentist, and this causes the rise of anxiety. Some patients feel humiliation or discomfort when dentists examine their mouths and inspect their gums and teeth. Anxiety can also arise from a narrow gap between the patient and the dentist during care. Also, a poor encounter with a previous dentist creates panic and leads to dental anxiety.

8. Verbal threats and incorrect sources of information: This is anxiety development by acquiring knowledge from other people and having prejudice in the dental community by dental phobic peers, derogatory societal connotations (e.g., the internet, and movies), and friends with unpleasant personal encounters. People are also profoundly influenced by what they see and hear in the news media. Indirect interactions can trigger fear. One way to get dental anxiety is by thinking about someone else's terrible traumatic experience. Often motivation shared from relatives and friends may contribute to dental anxiety. When someone who has had a poor dental experience describes what they had to experience, others may develop fear and dread dental appointments.

Signs of Dental anxiety

Anxiety may arise spontaneously, which ranges from apparent fear to intense panic. When dental anxiety is severe, it results in excessive panic and total avoidance of dental visits. The capacity to cope with a certain degree of pain ranges from person to person. Signs of dental fear differ from person to person. There are, however, sure signs and symptoms that could be observed generally. They include:

- Being detached from the dental environment and wanting to escape: An individual with dental anxiety often desires to escape the dental area. They want to get out and run. The essential explanations for this sign are environmental factors; the sound of handpieces and machines might generate panic and ignite the desire to escape. Many people with dental anxieties frequently postpone dental appointments because they distrust dental environments. Some people are quickly annoyed by the scent of the dental office or the dentist and their equipment.

- Panic expressed through shaking: Shaking is a typical physical symptom that one may encounter as part of one's dental anxiety. Dental anxiety can be identified through abnormal physical movements. When you are in an anxiety-provoking condition, the hormone epinephrine (also known as adrenaline) will be released to the body. Epinephrine transfers your blood to your skeletal muscles. You can also feel a rise in heart rate, and so the anxiety plays out. Some people are unable to find composure as they continue to fidget at the sight of dental instruments.

- Rapid breathing and shortness of breath: shortness of breath is one symptom of dental anxiety. At the sight of dental instruments or the dentist, one could feel tightness in the chest or struggle to breathe. One can also be hyperventilated (fast breathing) due to phobia at the sight of a dentist. When a person is nervous, their breathing can be disturbed. Panic will increase the respiratory rate and cause other health problems.

- Lack of concentration and Crying: Hormones control how our body functions, and as anxiety creeps in, our body reacts inappropriately. Worry will create a loss of focus. Dental anxiety may be cause for concern and exhaustion. It affects the pace and ability of the brain and can contribute to confusion. This symptom is often seen among infants and teens who cannot tolerate dentists and dental equipment. Some people demonstrate their distress by either screaming or throwing a tantrum. Some patients fail to pay attention because of their fear and thinking that dental operations would hurt.

- Sweating profusely and stammering: Dental anxiety may trigger a lack of confidence to talk in certain people. They wouldn't be free enough to provide the required information. People appear to display their anxiety whenever they cannot speak and clarify thoroughly to the dentist and explain what is wrong. Sweat is linked to fear. It usually hits you at once. If one is nervous, one can begin to sweat uncontrollably. Stuttering may also be a symptom of dental discomfort. The sight of a few instruments could make a stutter. Among some individuals, stuttering is so slight that others do not notice it at all. For a subset of individuals who are stuttering, the disorder can be so severe that it makes it very difficult to speak. When dental anxiety hits, stuttering and sweating can take the stage in a human.

- Having insomnia before the appointment: Sleep problems can be characterized as a disturbance in the quality and quantity of sleep due to certain irregularities. In a survey performed by Almoznino and Associates (2015), up to 50 percent of many who reported experiencing dental anxiety also revealed that they did not have enough sleep. Forty-five percent of survey respondents have said that they had used sleeping pills in the past. However, when 87 percent of survey respondents reported trusting the dentist, it is essential to demonstrate how powerful a dentist can be with their patients. Sleep conditions occur in different forms and affect an enormous number of people. Many individuals have dental anxieties right before their dental appointments, which resulted with lack of sleep. They remain frustrated to the extent where they could cancel their appointment.

These symptoms are evident and vary in different people. These signs occur before the date of appointment or on the day of the appointment. Some individuals who haven't had unpleasant dental encounters also develop phobia from listening to false dental trauma stories. They buy into the media stereotyping and find themselves resisting dental visits due to nervousness or anxiety. It is necessary to find a way to manage dental anxiety as it has consequences that may lead to extreme conditions.

Effects of dental anxiety

Bad decisions often result in bad consequences. Though it is more widely known that dental anxiety has highly detrimental effects on oral and general health, dental anxiety also has the most significant effects on an individual's medical, social, psychological, and emotional well-being. Some of these effects may include but not limited to:

1. Psychological effect: Psychosocial effect is identified as the effect of biological and environmental factors on a person. The dental environment has a significant impact on individuals and can create anxiety in the atmosphere. The psychological

impact of dental anxiety can include signs of and reactions to fear. Often, one of these symptoms is cardiac racing, which may lead to heart failure in adults and a variety of panic attacks. A few people express a feeling of exhaustion following a dental consultation to the point that they can still not handle regular day-to-day tasks. This will continue for a while until they have completely recovered from their anxiety. Some psychological effects are negative feelings. This happens before the date of the appointment. There may be an uneasy feeling that something might go wrong during the course of the appointment. People often worry about the pain before they even experience it; they are physically exhausted even before dental procedures begin. Dental anxiety can cause a person to overload the brain and mind, causing a lack of psychological balance.

2. Cognitive effect: Cognitive effects frequently begin gradually but advance until they substantially hinder the quality of life of the affected individual. Dental anxiety is commonly manifested as changes in patterns of thought or material. Without proper dental check-ups, one may have a toothache that can ultimately lead to dental damage. Tooth loss may trigger neurotransmitters in the brain. Teeth are linked to other organs in the body by nerves that assist in sensory processing and spatial awareness. The teeth are associated with areas of the brain. Tooth loss can lead to changes in the actual brain or mood fluctuations. Dental anxiety can also lead to a loss of sleep for a very long time. Many people sit awake for days or weeks before their appointment. Those suffering from dental anxiety from lack of sleep due to worry, which may lead to inactivity in their everyday activities.

3. Behavioral effect: There are typical indicators of fear that people encounter regarding emotions, attitudes, perceptions, and physical experiences regarding dental appointments. Dental phobia is capable of influencing one's actions. Fear of getting close to the dentist's office or dental clinic can contribute to such behaviors. Behavioral consequences of dental anxiety can include violence, hypervigilance anxiety disorders, intrusive behavioral disorders, or reactive aggression. Hypervigilance is a form of cognitive alertness. When one is in a situation of hypervigilance, they are highly alert to your environment. It will make one feel sensitive to any unknown threats, either from other humans or the setting. Sometimes, many of these reactions are exaggerated. Dental anxiety sets you up for aggressive reactions, and it may lead to irrational behaviour. Dental anxiety is capable of escalating both physical and emotional response. One can also be mentally detached and suffer bouts of depression or erratic behavior of emotion. The phobia may go as far as having an impact on quality of life. Dental anxiety will also generate fear of certain types of food such as hard foods (due to a decreased ability to eat or avoid tooth decay), or frozen food (due to reactions). However, it may lead to positive impact in certain individuals who then decide to take their oral hygiene seriously. These individuals recognize the value of oral hygiene as a result of oral distress. However, it is still recommended to go for dental checkup because that will not replace professional care.

In contrast, most people are affected negatively by dental anxiety. Behavioral effects also include mitigation and other habits related to nutrition, oral hygiene, including self-medication. Some people go as far as taking medications that are not recommended by a specialist, which may cause more dental damage.

4. Health effect: Several studies have reported that people with dental phobia have more oral cavities and worse dental hygiene than others. This could be the product of missing visits with the dentist, bad oral hygiene, or bad brushing habits. It can be exacerbated by smoking, which induces gum disease, or by heavy sugar intake, which encourages cavities. High levels of anxiety can contribute to the avoidance of dental treatment, which can have adverse effects on one's oral health and quality of life. Oral hygiene and overall welfare could be in a more impoverished state as a result of dental distress. The significant effect of dental anxiety on general health is due to sleep disturbance and often heart issues and panic attacks. These sleep disturbances may affect everyday life and work practices. It can also lead to exhaustion. Sleep disruption is the product of overthinking, which may reduce the efficiency of one's daily activities. It may also result in unhealthy weight loss. In certain situations, dental anxiety may have severe effects such as diabetes, heart diseases, weak dentition, and poor oral hygiene. It is worth fighting dental distress to protect overall wellbeing.

5. Social effect: Dental well-being is closely tied to our social and mental welfare. Usually, we grin and show our teeth to everyone. When they're not in good condition and clean, our emotional and social well-being is affected. Poor dental care can significantly influence the performance of an individual in many ways, especially when it comes to eating, chatting,

and smiling. Dental problems prevent people from opening their mouths. And could have implications in some social environments. Broken or loose teeth often complicates chewing and feeding. Despite these issues, many patients with dental phobias are waiting for their suffering to become intolerable. Mental and dental well-being correlates each other as mental problems can lead to a lack of oral hygiene and vice versa, which can lead to social anxieties and low self-esteem. Research has found that even the side effects of inadequate oral hygiene may have a detrimental impact on behavioral and social health. This research has shown clearly that dental anxiety can influence people's professional lives and social connections.

The risk of not overcoming dental anxiety

It's fair to say that few individuals want to visit their dentist. When patients postpone their dental appointment for a long time, there is increase likelihood that the care provided when they chose to go will be complicated (root canal procedure, surgical removal etc). This is because if decay is not treated soon enough, it advances by destroying more dental tissue, gradually damaging the nerve in the tooth, and increasing the chance of disease. If this condition is left untreated it could result in teeth fracturing which may lead to teeth submerging under the gums, making removal challenging. For the patient, this also involves wasting more time in the dentist's chair and causing more discomfort following surgery. Delaying dental treatments will do more harm than good. Individuals who neglect careful treatment of their teeth by not visiting a dentist are not only at risk of contracting tooth and dental disease but are also at risk of developing infections and disorders in other areas of their bodies. Dentistry can have a significant impact on the overall well-being of the person, and neglect to professional care will cause several anomalies. Poor oral hygiene can contribute to odor in the mouth, which can have a considerable effect on one's social contact. Keeping good teeth and gums is a long-term task. The sooner you develop the correct oral hygiene habits like cleaning, flossing, and minimizing sugar intake, the better it is to prevent expensive dental treatments and long-term health complications. The more you neglect dental appointments, the more harmful the result will be, and the more reason to visit the dental clinic. You're not expected to wait until you get signs to see the dentist. Visiting the dentist would typically allow them to spot a problem before you have the symptoms. If you have any early signs of oral health complications, you should try to resolve oral anxieties and make an appointment with the dentist as the prevention of oral diseases is best.

CHAPTER 3
Oral health

> *"Oral health is just as important as getting regular exercise. It's not just about getting a cavity filled; it's about the overall health of the individual – Jennifer Williams."*

Oral health involves the cleansing of the oral cavity in the broader context, whether at home or a clinical level. Oral health can also be referred to as oral hygiene. It is an essential component to the overall health. A healthy mouth encourages you to chat, laugh, smell, taste, touch, eat, and express various feelings confidently without any physical discomfort. This is vital to your well-being. Oral hygiene is a primary predictor of general health and excellent standards of living. The responsibility and consequences of poor oral hygiene are enormous. Without good oral care, it can be challenging to live a happy life. Lack of adequate oral hygiene leads to dental disorders and other cavity-related diseases.

Moreover, it can adversely affect one's relationships, professional interactions, social life, and physical health. Naturally, the first thing people encounter when they see you is your face and teeth. Every good smile makes a very good impression. Caring well for your mouth is a worthwhile pursuit. Healthy oral and dental hygiene can help avoid bad breath (halitosis), tooth loss, and gum disease. It helps maintain your teeth as you grow older. Your teeth are entitled to get cleaner and healthier. You feel better about yourself as you take proper care of them. Better teeth and healthier gums only contribute to a happier life. A good smile takes you far. A healthy mouth ensures that one is free from dangerous bacteria, and in some cases parasites, that can spread from the gum to teeth and infect the whole body.

Dental problems

Oral diseases are dental problems. Everyone is likely to experience dental issues sometime in their life. We make use of our mouths and teeth every day, so dental issues may be unavoidable over one's life span. Oral problems are often the product of inadequate or insufficient dental care. Many dental issues can be avoided as a result of good oral hygiene. According to the World Health Organization, approximately 60 to 90 percent of children in schools have had at least one oral cavity. Nearly 100 percent of adults have had at least one dental cavity.

In contrast, around 15 and 20 percent of the adult population between the ages of 35 and 44 have severe gum disease. About 30 percent of people across the globe between 65 and 74 have no natural teeth left. Some of these dental issues that contribute to these complications include:

- Tooth caries: tooth caries can also be called cavities or tooth decay. Tooth decay occurs as a result of the bacteria that cause decay. As decay-causing bacteria make contact with carbohydrates and sugar from food and drinks, they form an acid. This acid will damage the enamel of the tooth, causing it to lose its materials. It can happen if one eats or drinks foods and beverages containing mainly sugar and starchy carbs. The combined effects of these "acid strikes" will allow the enamel to begin to lose its substance. These bacteria produce acids that attack your tooth and lead to a crack or rotting of your tooth. The breaks in the tooth are called a cavity, and it can lead to discomfort, pain, and severe distress. Tooth cavity is an infectious disease which evolves step by step! The first step is the destruction of the enamel, which can go on painlessly. At this stage, your dentist tells you that you have a cavity. Most patients usually ignore it because they say, "I don't feel anything." The second stage is the process in which the dentin is targeted. At this stage, the discomfort starts to occur, but mostly after consuming spicy, cold or sweet food. The dental pulp is attacked at the third stage, causing intense pain. At this stage, the pain is intense enough that most people can't sleep through it. The fourth stage, which is the last stage, is marked by an abscess in the teeth and extremely severe pain. During this final phase, germs will contaminate the blood and trigger other pathologies at a distance. In general, cavities can do considerable harm to your teeth. In addition to discomfort, it can be the cause of the degradation of the dental pulp or general sepsis in the patient's body. Anybody can suffer tooth decay. If it's not properly taken care of, it can lead to tooth loss.

- Gum diseases: An example of gum disorders is gingivitis, irritation of the gums. It's typically the product of bacteria forming around your teeth due to improper brushing and flossing practices. Gingivitis can cause your gums to swell and bleed while you brush or floss. If proper care is not taken, gingivitis can result in periodontitis, a more severe infection. This is more extreme and can potentially lead to a loss of teeth. Gingivitis signs include swollen and puffy gums that bleed quickly when a person cleans his/hers teeth. An individual with gingivitis can also recover with proper oral hygiene, such as longer, more regular brushing, and flossing. And sometimes adding antibacterial mouthwash can help. In some cases of gum disease, patients do not even know that they have gingivitis, though there may be minor symptoms such as bleeding. However, the condition must be closely monitored and treated immediately. Adults with periodontitis should visit the dentist more regularly to avoid excessive bone loss.

- Cracked tooth: Cracked teeth can occur through chewing on hard food, grinding your teeth, and may also arise as you age. One may suffer from damaged teeth due to several problems that may be either dental grinding pressure or large fillings that limit the quality of the teeth. Also, chewing or scraping hard food, such as nuts or hard candy, or accidental blows to the mouth can cause cracked teeth.

- Examples of other dental/oral complications include a sore or ulcer, pain in your mouth, face or chin, chewing discomfort, a distorted sense of taste, or a sour taste in your lips and bad breath. Some of these may be related to other health problems.

Causes of dental problems

Our oral cavity contains all manner of bacteria, viruses, and fungi. Some make up the usual flora of your mouth. Because the mouth is a gateway to the body, they are usually harmless in limited amounts. But a high-sugar diet produces situations in which acid-producing bacteria can thrive.

Most dental problems are caused purely by our actions. These practices include:

1. Inadequate brushing and flossing habits: you could still acquire a dental problem even though you clean your teeth regularly. There are many reasons why, even after cleaning your teeth, they're still going to be bad. One of the most common causes is not using the right toothpaste and toothbrush. Both are critical to your oral health, as they have vast effects on your smile. It is essential to choose the right toothpaste. The ADA recommends fluoride toothpaste. One should clean one's teeth at least twice a day and floss effectively. It is advisable to brush first thing in the morning and at night after dinner.

2. Frequent feeding on sugary snacks and beverages: Sugar will hurt your teeth, especially when you chew, sugars in food and drinks are combined with oral bacteria to make plaque. It's a toxic, acidic material that surrounds your teeth with the aim of destroying the tooth enamel. The more sugary substance you eat, the more plaque your mouth produces, and the more cavities you get. Chewing sugar-filled gums and consuming sugar-coated cakes and sweets will cause tooth decay and oral damage. If you're drinking sugary drinks every day, there's a strong likelihood that you will develop a dental problem. It is clinically proven that an increase in sugar intake increases the amount of cavities. People with a "sweet tooth" have more cavities— even when they brush more frequently. To tackle dental problems, keep your consumption of high-sugar foods and drinks to a reasonable level, especially between meals and right before bedtime.

Proper care of your teeth and adopting a healthier lifestyle are the easiest ways to win the fight against tooth decay.

3. Genetic reasons: Dental problems can exist in the family. The cause of dental issues may be found in one's genome. Many oral health disorders are inherited. This means that you could be at greater risk of contracting some diseases, despite your practices. It may also be transmitted as a result of poor general oral hygiene. With so many possible complications that can be passed on, maintaining your oral health is not simple. Still, you wouldn't have to do it independently. Make sure you see the dentist regularly.

How to maintain proper dental hygiene

Prevention is the secret to keeping your mouth healthy. Proper oral care helps you live a safe, long, and pain-free life. To maintain healthy teeth, it's crucial to start setting up a proper oral care regimen early and stick to it all your life. Most of the dental problems may be avoided by paying closer attention to prevention. If you want to have healthy dentition and a wonderful smile, it is crucial to clean the whole mouth carefully every day. To maintain proper dental hygiene, one should:

- Clean their teeth after each meal: It is beneficial to rinse first and then brush for 2-3 minutes to clear bacterial plaque from the surfaces of your teeth and gums and eliminate any food traces. It is preferable to use a toothbrush fitted with soft bristles with a medium-small head to penetrate even the most challenging areas of the mouth effectively. Also, it is ideal to change the toothbrush at least once every two months.

- Brush one arch at a time: this is the best way to ensure successful washing. Don't neglect the inner areas of the teeth, which are more challenging to access and clean, but equally important.

- It is recommended to brush the exterior and inner surfaces, to eliminate the bacterial plaque that causes inflammation to the gums.

- Using regular dental floss to extract bacterial plaque interproximally from places not reachable by the toothbrush bristles. Dental floss can be used at least once a day, usually at night. Pay attention to proper use: it is not enough to insert it between the teeth and move it back and forth, but it is necessary to embrace the tooth and to slip the floss from the gum upwards and vice versa, with decisive motions but without causing harm to the gums.

- According to the ADA, fluoride toothpaste is preferred: it makes the enamel more robust. It helps protect it from the demineralizing activity of the bacterial plaque acids.

- Practice a balanced, sugar-low diet. High sugar diets favor the development of bacteria and, subsequently, the creation of cavities. In general, it is helpful to eat a nutritious diet rich in fruits and vegetables; these foods contain essential vitamins and minerals (vitamins C, A, and D, calcium, phosphorus, potassium, sodium, iron, and magnesium) to protect your teeth, keep your gums safe, and boost your immune defenses.

- Carry out periodic checks, at least every six months, to properly assess the health of the mouth and deeply extract the residual plaque and tartar through regular cleaning activity.

Home oral hygiene is not enough to thoroughly remove bacterial plaque and tartar. You must also regularly schedule a visit to the dentist. Also, during the visit, it will be possible to conduct a comprehensive examination to detect potential problems that, if handled in time, will prevent any issues relating to the oral cavity of an individual.

CHAPTER 4
Dental visitations

Expectations vs. reality

Dental appointments are scheduled visits to the dental clinic. It's a vital component of maintaining the health and well-being of your smile, and overall health.

Many people feel that dental visits are not required. Certain myths rule and ruin reality. Chances are you've heard a lot of dental misconceptions in your lifetime. These myths and expectations are one sole cause of dental anxiety. These beliefs may over-exaggerate or distort the reality about the specifics of the dental procedure and can result in a patient being afraid of dental visits. Patients who may need adequate dental work risk their well-being by missing dental appointments. Most stereotypes are the product of misunderstanding or misinterpretation of the system. In a dental office environment, a patient may encounter a lack of interaction from the dentist and may believe that the dentist is not caring or insensitive to their concerns. As a result of these myths, many perceive dental visitations to be unpleasant and not deserving of their time and effort.

Many dental anxiety patients' perceptions of dental appointments are typically far from the reality since their assumptions are the product of anxiety. Some misconceptions include:

That dentists are usually terrifying, severe, and not necessarily attentive to patient needs. They feel that dentists are not compassionate enough to treat teeth because they don't feel the discomfort. They also believe like the dentist is unable to work with patients who have a dental phobia or extreme fear about medication.

- The truth is that many dentists are qualified people, who understand the plight of their patient. I am a dentist and I have dental anxiety. Medical treatment is part of the job requirement of any dentist. Their willingness to help you feel relaxed and secure makes their jobs much easier. They can offer as much support and as many resources as you need to help feel relaxed. The only difference here is that individual personalities differ which can contribute to some misconceptions. Some people fear that the dentist will criticize them and that the dentist might also speak ill of them and their lack of oral hygiene. Others believe the dentist may be insincere about the condition of their teeth.

  The reality remains that, as experts, dentists can do all they can to get their message out in a manner that everybody would appreciate. They try not to instill anxiety in the patient and deliberately choose their terms. Dentists are qualified medical practitioners who frequently witness the most severe conditions with bad oral health. It is more than likely that they have seen cases more severe than yours. A dentist is qualified to work with your complaints in a competent way. You can trust them with your dental problems! Many times, I get patients who apologize for not cleaning their teeth before they came. That is not a problem— dentists' CLEAN teeth!

- People claim that there should be no dental appointment until there is a dental problem. They assume that a dental appointment is not required if the teeth look very healthy. Many people attend the dentist only when there is a problem, and others do not because they doubt the results of dental visits. They foresee disastrous results from dental appointments, so they don't bother to make appointments. Many dental issues may not be felt by a patient until they have become severe. A dental visit is mandatory for all. Consistent checks are essential to ensure proper oral health.

- Another misconception is that all dental operations are unpleasant, and their pain lasts for a very long time. Some believe that having needles in the gums is going to be extremely painful. Some say that dental operations and experiences cause extreme discomfort during the process. These are simply not true and vary from one individual to another. Also, technology has advanced, and many dental procedures no longer leave a person in excruciating pain. Dentists use several methods and techniques strategies to reduce the patient's reaction to pain. Patients can also take analgesics before the treatment. New advances in dental technologies also offer excellent alternatives to debilitating injection methods. Machines and tools are closely handled by the dentist. The teeth and gum are sensitive parts of the mouth which must be treated with caution. Dental services are designed to enable you to live free from dental complications. Besides, not all dental conditions require dental surgery. Some people just need a checkup or a prescription. Dental treatments will never be done with the intention of hurting you.

- There is a misconception that preserving good dental hygiene is difficult, and it is not compulsory to see a dentist on a regular basis; some also conclude that dental procedures cost a lot and are not affordable.

The truth of the matter is maintaining good oral hygiene is not for the wealthy, but for everybody. It needs one's dedication and intentionality. Dental care is given for everyone, and dental clinics are not only made for the affluent or the elderly. Proper oral care begins with you and ends with a dental appointment. Maintaining good dental hygiene is not complicated, but it requires one to be vigilant. Brushing twice a day with the correct technique, keeping a balanced diet, and flossing daily are essential steps in oral hygiene. Following these measures with routine dental check-ups will guarantee that the teeth are in outstanding condition.

Dental appointments are very significant. You will feel outstanding about your general well-being if you take dental health seriously. The quality of your smile is essential, and the dentist will help to keep your smile healthy and beautiful. Ask your dentist to teach and show you how to brush your teeth. Everything should be learned properly—including brushing. Also, dental appointments can be made anytime you're comfortable; you will need to contact an available dentist.

Why people should visit the dentist

People believe they need to see a dentist only when they have a toothache. However, this is not the case; visiting a dentist is as critical as consuming a healthy diet. You should choose the right dentist of your choice. Dental checkups are necessary for preserving safe teeth and gums. The dentist will not just check for cavities during the appointment. Other components of the exam include the gums and the mouth; this is to ensure that there is general health in the oral cavity.

Oral cancer screening is part of dental checkup. Many diseases often start with the mouth. Sometimes cavities cannot be avoided. Even people with excellent oral hygiene may have holes, tartar, or plaque. Going to the dentist is also effective in keeping those things under control. Caries are the diseases of the teeth that make the tissues worse. If ignored, caries can begin to migrate to the interior of the tooth, producing abscesses, cysts, and granulomas.

> Plaque, too, should not be ignored. It's a material that collects on the top of the teeth. It is quickly dissolved, and the dentist will inform you whether it is there or not. However, if it is not eliminated, the plaque mineralizes, creating calculus. It is a lot tougher to get rid of calculus because it is a harder material. A professional cleaning is essential to prevent calculus build up.

A. Visiting for oral cancer checks: Oral cancer is a severe condition. It may become fatal without early detection. Fortunately, it is also easy to handle if detected easily. It is also helpful to go to the dentist to monitor the onset of this condition; if it is not detected early it may make the situation worse. The oral cancer screening is painless and non- destructive.

B. Keeping unhealthy oral behavior under control: Many terrible practices can hurt oral health. Chewing ice, biting your nails, clenching your jaw, grinding your teeth, vigorously brushing your teeth, or smoking are some of the bad habits that can inflict harm. People often don't realize the problems they are creating. Many of our everyday practices are harmful to our teeth. Going to the dentist also helps to recognize the issues and conditions they trigger. Some behaviors can sound harmless, but they can inflict damage on your teeth.

Visiting a dentist will help us put a stop to any bad practices and reduce bad decisions.

C. Some other advantages of dental visitation is helping with bad breath, which may impair social experiences and partnerships. Other procedures may include teeth whitening, fillings that replicate the look of real teeth, tooth repair, and full smile make-up.

When should we visit the dentist?

Dental visitation is absolutely life-saving, as you look out for all aspects of your life. Dental fear deters you from taking responsibility for the management of your teeth. Dental anxiety can also rob you of oral health and overall well-being. Many people plan to see the dentist, but they don't know when. It is necessary not to procrastinate or treat dental appointments with levity. Dental visitation should be taken seriously.

Today, modern dentistry has taken significant steps forward. A comparatively small portion of the population is on a prophylaxis and regular appointment. However, some people still feel that if the teeth don't hurt, a dentist's appointment is a waste of time and resources. The number of people that visit the dentist regularly is increasing. The frequency at which it is vital to go to a dentist varies depending on the person and their oral health. For individuals with good oral hygiene, two visits a year are appropriate. Others may need to go at least every three months. Preventive care, as a standard, does not take a lot of time. As a general rule, every person should visit their dentist every six months. For those who are more vulnerable to periodontal issues, on the other hand, it might be essential to have their mouth checked, and their teeth cleaned more regularly. You and your dentist should establish your standard of care. Your dentist is in a position to assess the optimal amount of the meetings. It is important to keep up with one's appointments.

The basic scheme for healthy individuals is twice a year, but as disease or pathology increases, the number of visits increase. It is advised that an assessment be carried out every three months. This system is also applicable to children. Daily visits to the same doctor enables babies to get used to the doctor and to experience him or her without terror and fear.

Managing dental anxiety during dental appointments

It has been documented that 8 out of 10 people have dental anxieties on or before dental appointments. There are a variety of approaches to tackle dental anxiety. However, this dental distress can be treated and monitored with or without the help of the dentist. You may use a variety of strategies to ease anxiety and comfortably undergo dental tests and treatments. Here are a few techniques:

    a. Speak up, express your worries: Communication is also necessary for dental procedures. It's important to remember that expressing your emotions makes a lot of difference. If you're nervous or worried, inform the dentist and the staff of your fear. When you make your appointment, tell the staff that you're worried about dental appointments. Share any negative encounters that you might have had in the past, and ask for advice on coping mechanisms. Don't be scared to ask your questions. Speak to your dentist about discomfort when it starts, because your dentist knows how to work with you and make it more convenient. Being aware of what is going to happen often relieves one's worries of the unexpected. Don't let fear deprive you of a proper dental check-up.

b. Focus on gently breathing during dental procedures: When fear hits the air, one's heart starts to beat faster, and anxiety takes over. Breathing heavily and causing pressure to impair your breathing rate will lead to various other health complications, such as fainting and heart attacks. Often try to breathe gently and catch your breath during dental visitations and oral treatment. Track your breathing, focus on breathing gently, and be conscious. Relaxation begins with the subconscious. Use deep breathing exercises to help relieve muscle stress.

Count your breaths. Slowly inhale and then exhale with the same amount of counts. Do this five times when you're waiting for your appointment, or after a break while you're seated in a dental chair.

c. Listen to relaxing music: Having your mind off the appointment can sound complicated when you're anxious, but some things may help you divert your thoughts. Some songs are soothing and relaxing. Certain music will take your mind away from dental anxiety. If you're bothered by the sound, carry your headphones so that you can listen to your favorite songs or audiobook.

d. Choose a convenient appointment time: It's essential to pick a low-stress appointment time. This helps to relieve discomfort and discomfort that may contribute to dental anxiety. When it's time to schedule dental appointments either as a new or existing patient, keep various things in mind. We just want our time invested effectively, and so does the dentist. Clear your work schedule on the time and date your appointment schedule. Make sure you feel comfortable.

e. Distract yourself and make yourself busy: When waiting for dental care, you should calm your mind and be distracted by reading a book or reading dental charts and entertaining visuals. Some dental offices have televisions. You may also fill your hands by holding a tension ball or playing with a small hand-held item like a fidget spinner. You can also imagine or visualize yourself on a relaxing seaside or in a garden.

f. Schedule your appointment with a pleasant dentist for yourself: They are always conscious and accommodating; they also understand what works for you. Read reviews and ask your friends, family, and neighbors which dentist they go to. In this age of social media, finding a good dentist is easier than ever before.

The next big thing for the people who visit the dentist

There are some advantages involved with dental visitations that can impede your dental anxiety. Everyone who wishes to live a healthy life should always take oral hygiene seriously. People who see dental hygiene as a priority have an advantage over people who do not see oral hygiene to be essential. Many of these benefits include the following:

1. One of the advantages of routine dental visits is that the dentist is easily able to detect problems that may eventually transform into more significant issues along the line. For example, a tiny cavity or some form of gum disease can be treated immediately. Frequent visits to the dentist have the benefit of identifying and resolving dental problems quickly. They also avoid potential oral complications and health concerns.

2. Another benefit is that good dental hygiene would preserve their teeth. Healthy teeth can be a mark of beauty for great opportunities at work when white teeth shine. Shiny teeth enhance positive perceptions about a person. These people also may be more open to friendships and relationships.

3. Dental visitation helps create confidence. Many who frequent the dentist still have strong faith in themselves and their teeth. They live with unfailing self-belief, and they are so sure of themselves everywhere and at any moment. Their smiles are radiant, too.

4. Getting dental pain or worries about your oral health could cause you sleepless nights. Dental health gives peace of mind to those who take dental appointments seriously. Visiting a dentist and protecting yourself from dental complications will keep your mental stability.

5. People who visit dentists are willing to share positive news about dental care and how dentists behave with their patients.

They will be encouraged to share their experiences, and their lives would become a testimony of standard oral hygiene. Taking dental appointments seriously will improve the quality of your life.

CHAPTER 5
The Dentist's Corner

The essential duties of the dentist involve the protection of the teeth. After a tentative consultation to gather the patient's medical records and to verify the state of health of the oral cavity, the dentist plans an action plan to be performed and recommends the appropriate procedures, depending on the situation. Typically, X-ray radiographs are used in the diagnostic process to demonstrate illnesses, pathogens, dental and jaw malformations. The dentist then performs the negotiated procedures with the chair assistant; it is standard procedure to prescribe local anesthetics to patients to reduce the discomfort encountered during the process. The most critical methods undertaken by the dentist include the cleaning of the plaque and calculus, the filling and treatment of dental caries, the restoration of the chipped or missing teeth, the replacement and devitalization of the teeth, the repair of root canals, and the insertion of dental prostheses. Drugs and antibiotics may be recommended if required for treatment.

Another very critical role of the dentist is the instructional component. During the appointments, the dentist tells the patient about proper oral hygiene habits, the use of toothbrushes, toothpaste, and dental floss. The patient may receive the guidance of the dental hygienist, the treatment of dental equipment, and implants. The dentist's responsibilities may include carrying out numerous administrative and legal tasks relating to the collection, recording, and storing of medical reports and the maintenance of patient health data, with the help of the dental office's delegate.

Also, it is the dentist's responsibility to recognize and support patients with dental anxiety. The dentist learns various successful ways to cope with stress and what drugs to use for certain cases of dental anxiety.

Effective ways to handle patients with dental anxiety

There are some methods used by dentists to ease anxiety in patients. As a dentist, you should employ:

a. Clear and easy communication: Dentists attempt to make the patient feel comfortable in a dental environment. They have calm conversations and listen to the patient carefully. Often, the dentist assures that there is sufficient comprehension and no discomfort in the room. They try to understand the patients point of view in an effort to serve the patient better.

b. Usage of laughing gas: nitrous oxide can allow patients to relax during dental treatment. The mask is attached to the patients' faces, and they breathe in a combination of oxygen and nitrous oxide. It will take effect in a few minutes and will wear off rapidly. The patient will be awake and calm. They will be able to communicate with dentists. But pain is usually eased off (especially on children).

c. Using medications: Usage oral anxiety-relieving (anxiolytic) drugs (such as diazepam) are often administered by dentists or clinicians to help nervous patients cope. A short-acting, thin, single dose is usually given one hour before a dental appointment. Medication can only be issued after consultation with the dentist or specialist.

d. Conscious anesthesia: This form of sedation includes obtaining drugs by a drip inserted in the vein of the hand or arm. A dentist gives intravenous (IV) sedation with specialized anesthesia training). It may be done in a dentist clinic with extra facilities or in a hospital. Patients become comfortable and typically fall asleep, but they would respond to instructions. The dentists would only use anesthesia when it is required.

General anesthetics can be a suitable choice for certain individual patients. The anesthetist would still need to examine the patient before general anesthetics. However, this kind of treatment is not recommended for everyone. It is essential to choose a dentist that understands your level of anxiety so that they can be empathetic about your situation.

CONCLUSION

Fear is a human emotion that is caused by a potential threat. Dental anxiety is a dangerous condition since the consequences are extensive. It is important to remember that coping with your dental fears and overcoming your anxiety results in an award: wide-reaching well-being. Dental anxiety prevents good oral health. Poor oral hygiene stops you from laughing, smiling or even engaging in conversations. It tends to make one lose confidence, and one may not be able to communicate easily. Eventually, it could lead to depression, which may spiral down into bigger problems.

The dentist is not your enemy, they want the best for you, and they are willing to help you. Dental visits are for everyone— not a few chosen ones. The dentist is your friend; they want to ensure that your smile and dental health are up to standard. If you go to the dentist regularly, you may eliminate significant concerns that could resolve to more panic and anxiety. Going to the dentist should be a protective step to live better and improve the quality of life. Write your thoughts down, be ready to talk to the dentist and the staff about any issues you might have.

Finally, we need your mouth to make the world a better place. Your dental health is what defines your smile, and dental anxiety hides your smile.

A mouth that expresses greatness and spreads positivity is a mouth that is well cared for.

www.ingramcontent.com/pod-product-compliance
Lightning Source LLC
Chambersburg PA
CBHW031502210526
45463CB00003B/1040